EASY DIABETIC COOKBOOK FOR BEGINNERS

BEGINNERS

Simple Recipes for Delicious & Nutritious Meals

T. John

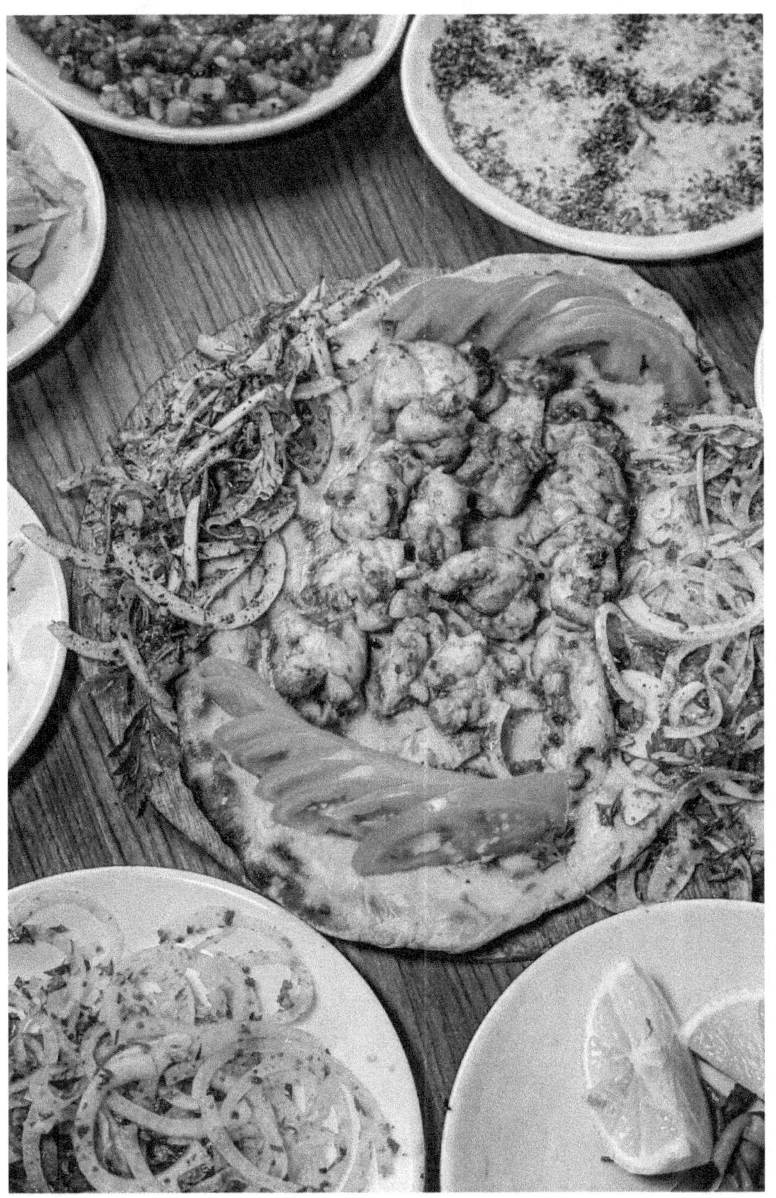

TABLE OF CONTENTS

Chapter 6: Desserts 97

Chapter 7: Smoothies 115

INTRODUCTION

I magine you're driving a car. Your body is the engine, and glucose is the fuel it runs on. In diabetes, something throws a wrench in the system. Either your body doesn't make enough insulin, the key that unlocks the door for glucose to enter your cells, or your cells become resistant to it. The result? A traffic jam of sugar in your bloodstream, honking its horn in the form of fatigue, thirst, and even blurry vision.

But despair not, fellow motorist! Just like you wouldn't throw random junk into your engine, you can manage your diabetes by choosing the right fuel – a delicious, diabetic-friendly diet. Think of it as a gourmet road trip through the five food groups, with each bite keeping your blood sugar purring like a well-tuned engine.

First stop: Veggies and Fruits. These vibrant roadsigns guide you towards a cornucopia of vitamins, minerals, and fiber – the traffic cops that keep your system humming. Load up on leafy greens, colorful peppers, juicy berries, and don't forget the humble tomato – a champion of lycopene, a powerful antioxidant. Remember, moderation is key, so portion control is your GPS, helping you navigate between a light snack and a filling meal.

Next up: Whole Grains. Ditch the white bread and refined carbs – they're like sugar rockets spiking your blood sugar levels. Instead, opt for whole-wheat bread, brown rice, quinoa, and oats – slow-burning fuel that keeps your energy tank steady throughout the day. Think of them as the sturdy tires of your car, taking you the distance without a wobble.

Protein Powerhouse. Now, imagine your muscles as the engine pistons. They need protein to stay strong and resilient. Lean meats like chicken, fish, and beans are your pit stops for quality protein, while nuts and lentils offer a bonus of healthy fats and fiber. Just remember, portion sizes matter – think palm-sized servings for meat and a handful for nuts.

Don't forget the Dairy Detour! Calcium-rich dairy, like yogurt and cheese, strengthens your bones, another crucial part of your health journey. Choose low-fat options to keep your cholesterol in check. Think of it as adding shock absorbers to your car, smoothing out the bumps along the road.

Hydration Highway. Water is the lifeblood of your body, and especially important for managing diabetes. Ditch sugary drinks and fill your thermos with plain water, sparkling water with a squeeze of citrus, or unsweetened herbal teas. Water keeps your engine cool, flushes out toxins, and helps prevent dehydration, a common diabetes symptom.

Remember, the diabetic-friendly diet is not a restrictive one-way street. It's a vibrant, winding road filled with delicious pit stops and breathtaking scenery. Explore new flavors, experiment with spices, and discover hidden gems like chia seeds and avocado. With a little planning and creativity, you can turn your diet into a culinary adventure, keeping your blood sugar in check and your taste buds tingling with delight.

So, buckle up, grab your healthy snacks, and embark on your delicious journey towards a well-managed diabetes. Remember, you're the driver, and with the right choices, you can cruise through life feeling energized, empowered, and ready to savor every bite!

Chapter 1: 30 Day Meal Plan

Week 1:

Day 1:

- Breakfast: Nutty Oatmeal Delight
- Lunch: Grilled Chicken Salad with Lemon Vinaigrette
- Dinner: Baked Cod with Lemon and Herbs
- Snack: Hummus and Veggie Sticks
- Dessert: Sugar-Free Chocolate Avocado Mousse

Day 2:

- Breakfast: Veggie-Packed Omelette
- Lunch: Quinoa and Black Bean Stuffed Peppers
- Dinner: Eggplant Lasagna
- Snack: Cheese and Grape Skewers
- Dessert: Berry and Greek Yogurt Popsicles

Day 3:

- Breakfast: Greek Yogurt Parfait
- Lunch: Turkey and Avocado Wrap

- Dinner: Cilantro Lime Chicken
- Snack: Cucumber and Cream Cheese Bites
- Dessert: Almond Flour Pumpkin Muffins

Day 4:

- Breakfast: Berry Blast Smoothie Bowl
- Lunch: Lentil and Vegetable Soup
- Dinner: Quinoa and Spinach Stuffed Mushrooms
- Snack: Edamame with Sea Salt
- Dessert: Dark Chocolate Covered Strawberries

Day 5:

- Breakfast: Avocado and Turkey Wrap
- Lunch: Shrimp and Quinoa Bowl
- Dinner: Turkey and Sweet Potato Skillet
- Snack: Almond and Cranberry Energy Bites
- Dessert: Lemon Chia Seed Pudding

Day 6:

- Breakfast: Quinoa Breakfast Casserole
- Lunch: Caprese Salad with Balsamic Glaze
- Dinner: Lemon Garlic Shrimp with Zoodles

- Snack: Avocado Salsa with Whole Grain Chips
- Dessert: Baked Apple with Cinnamon

Day 7:

- Breakfast: Spinach and Feta Scramble
- Lunch: Chickpea and Vegetable Stir-Fry
- Dinner: Asian-Inspired Salmon
- Snack: Greek Yogurt and Berries Parfait
- Dessert: Avocado Chocolate Pudding

Week 2:

Day 8:

- Breakfast: Whole Grain Pancakes with Berries
- Lunch: Salmon and Asparagus Foil Pack
- Dinner: Cauliflower and Chickpea Curry
- Snack: Roasted Red Pepper and Feta Dip
- Dessert: Coconut Flour Blueberry Bars

Day 9:

- Breakfast: Chia Seed Pudding
- Lunch: Zucchini Noodles with Pesto
- Dinner: Grilled Vegetable Medley

- Snack: Apple Slices with Peanut Butter
- Dessert: Pistachio and Cherry Frozen Yogurt

Day 10:

- Breakfast: Apple Cinnamon Steel-Cut Oats
- Lunch: Greek Chicken Pita
- Dinner: Balsamic Glazed Chicken Thighs
- Snack: Caprese Kabobs
- Dessert: Raspberry Almond Tart

Day 11:

- Breakfast: Smoked Salmon Bagel Stack
- Lunch: Cauliflower Fried Rice
- Dinner: Zesty Lemon Dill Tilapia
- Snack: Spicy Roasted Chickpeas
- Dessert: Vanilla Bean Panna Cotta

Day 12:

- Breakfast: Sweet Potato Hash with Eggs
- Lunch: Tuna Salad Lettuce Wraps
- Dinner: Ratatouille with Brown Rice
- Snack: Nut Mix with Dried Fruit

- Dessert: Mixed Berry Sorbet

Day 13:

- Breakfast: Cottage Cheese and Fruit Bowl
- Lunch: Turkey and Vegetable Skewers
- Dinner: Turkey Chili
- Snack: Guacamole with Jicama Slices
- Dessert: Pumpkin Pie Smoothie

Day 14:

- Breakfast: Almond Butter Banana Toast
- Lunch: Spinach and Mushroom Quesadilla
- Dinner: Spaghetti Squash Primavera
- Snack: Cottage Cheese and Pineapple Cups
- Dessert: Walnut and Date Energy Balls

Week 3:

Day 15:

- Breakfast: Veggie Breakfast Burrito
- Lunch: Broccoli and Cheddar Stuffed Chicken Breast
- Dinner: Mexican Cauliflower Rice Bowl

- Snack: Tomato Basil Bruschetta
- Dessert: Grilled Peaches with Honey Drizzle

Day 16:

- Breakfast: Nutty Oatmeal Delight
- Lunch: Grilled Chicken Salad with Lemon Vinaigrette
- Dinner: Baked Cod with Lemon and Herbs
- Snack: Hummus and Veggie Sticks
- Dessert: Sugar-Free Chocolate Avocado Mousse

Day 17:

- Breakfast: Veggie-Packed Omelette
- Lunch: Quinoa and Black Bean Stuffed Peppers
- Dinner: Eggplant Lasagna
- Snack: Cheese and Grape Skewers
- Dessert: Berry and Greek Yogurt Popsicles

Day 18:

- Breakfast: Greek Yogurt Parfait
- Lunch: Turkey and Avocado Wrap
- Dinner: Cilantro Lime Chicken

- Snack: Cucumber and Cream Cheese Bites
- Dessert: Almond Flour Pumpkin Muffins

Day 19:

- Breakfast: Berry Blast Smoothie Bowl
- Lunch: Lentil and Vegetable Soup
- Dinner: Quinoa and Spinach Stuffed Mushrooms
- Snack: Edamame with Sea Salt
- Dessert: Dark Chocolate Covered Strawberries

Day 20:

- Breakfast: Avocado and Turkey Wrap
- Lunch: Shrimp and Quinoa Bowl
- Dinner: Turkey and Sweet Potato Skillet
- Snack: Almond and Cranberry Energy Bites
- Dessert: Lemon Chia Seed Pudding

Day 21:

- Breakfast: Quinoa Breakfast Casserole
- Lunch: Caprese Salad with Balsamic Glaze
- Dinner: Lemon Garlic Shrimp with Zoodles
- Snack: Avocado Salsa with Whole Grain Chips

- Dessert: Baked Apple with Cinnamon

Week 4:

Day 22:

- Breakfast: Spinach and Feta Scramble
- Lunch: Chickpea and Vegetable Stir-Fry
- Dinner: Asian-Inspired Salmon
- Snack: Greek Yogurt and Berries Parfait
- Dessert: Avocado Chocolate Pudding

Day 23:

- Breakfast: Whole Grain Pancakes with Berries
- Lunch: Salmon and Asparagus Foil Pack
- Dinner: Cauliflower and Chickpea Curry
- Snack: Roasted Red Pepper and Feta Dip
- Dessert: Coconut Flour Blueberry Bars

Day 24:

- Breakfast: Chia Seed Pudding
- Lunch: Zucchini Noodles with Pesto
- Dinner: Grilled Vegetable Medley
- Snack: Apple Slices with Peanut Butter

- Dessert: Pistachio and Cherry Frozen Yogurt

Day 25:

- Breakfast: Apple Cinnamon Steel-Cut Oats
- Lunch: Greek Chicken Pita
- Dinner: Balsamic Glazed Chicken Thighs
- Snack: Caprese Kabobs
- Dessert: Raspberry Almond Tart

Day 26:

- Breakfast: Smoked Salmon Bagel Stack
- Lunch: Cauliflower Fried Rice
- Dinner: Zesty Lemon Dill Tilapia
- Snack: Spicy Roasted Chickpeas
- Dessert: Vanilla Bean Panna Cotta

Day 27:

- Breakfast: Sweet Potato Hash with Eggs
- Lunch: Tuna Salad Lettuce Wraps
- Dinner: Ratatouille with Brown Rice
- Snack: Nut Mix with Dried Fruit
- Dessert: Mixed Berry Sorbet

Day 28:

- Breakfast: Cottage Cheese and Fruit Bowl
- Lunch: Turkey and Vegetable Skewers
- Dinner: Turkey Chili
- Snack: Guacamole with Jicama Slices
- Dessert: Pumpkin Pie Smoothie

Day 29:

- Breakfast: Almond Butter Banana Toast
- Lunch: Spinach and Mushroom Quesadilla
- Dinner: Spaghetti Squash Primavera
- Snack: Cottage Cheese and Pineapple Cups
- Dessert: Walnut and Date Energy Balls

Day 30:

- Breakfast: Veggie Breakfast Burrito
- Lunch: Broccoli and Cheddar Stuffed Chicken Breast
- Dinner: Mexican Cauliflower Rice Bowl
- Snack: Tomato Basil Bruschetta
- Dessert: Grilled Peaches with Honey Drizzle

Chapter 2: Breakfast Recipes

This chapter is designed to kickstart your mornings with delicious and diabetes-friendly breakfast options. Each recipe is carefully crafted with wholesome ingredients to ensure a nutritious start to your day.

Nutty Oatmeal Delight

Ingredients:

- 1/2 cup rolled oats
- 1 cup unsweetened almond milk
- 1 tablespoon chopped nuts (almonds, walnuts, or pecans)
- 1/2 teaspoon ground cinnamon
- 1/2 teaspoon vanilla extract
- 1 tablespoon sugar-free maple syrup

Instructions:

1. In a saucepan, combine rolled oats and almond milk.
2. Cook over medium heat, stirring frequently until the oats are tender.

3. Stir in chopped nuts, cinnamon, vanilla extract, and maple syrup.

4. Cook for an additional 2-3 minutes, ensuring the mixture is well combined.

5. Serve warm and enjoy!

Nutrition Information:

- Calories: 250
- Protein: 7g
- Carbohydrates: 40g
- Fat: 8g
- Fiber: 6g
- Sugar: 5g
- Portion Size: 1 serving

Veggie-Packed Omelette

Ingredients:

- 2 large eggs
- 1/4 cup diced bell peppers (assorted colors)
- 1/4 cup diced tomatoes
- 2 tablespoons diced onions
- 1/4 cup baby spinach

- Salt and pepper to taste
- 1 teaspoon olive oil

Instructions:

1. In a bowl, beat the eggs and season with salt and pepper.
2. Heat olive oil in a non-stick pan over medium heat.
3. Add onions, bell peppers, and tomatoes to the pan, sautéing until softened.
4. Pour beaten eggs over the vegetables, ensuring even distribution.
5. When the edges start to set, add spinach and fold the omelette in half.
6. Cook until the eggs are fully set.
7. Slide onto a plate and serve.

Nutrition Information:

- Calories: 180
- Protein: 12g
- Carbohydrates: 8g
- Fat: 11g
- Fiber: 2g

- Sugar: 4g
- Portion Size: 1 omelette

Greek Yogurt Parfait

Ingredients:

- 1/2 cup Greek yogurt (unsweetened)
- 1/4 cup fresh berries (blueberries, strawberries, or raspberries)
- 2 tablespoons chopped nuts (almonds or walnuts)
- 1 tablespoon honey (optional)

Instructions:

1. In a glass or bowl, layer Greek yogurt, fresh berries, and chopped nuts.
2. Repeat the layers until the container is filled.
3. Drizzle honey on top for added sweetness if desired.
4. Serve chilled and savor the delightful parfait.

Nutrition Information:

- Calories: 220
- Protein: 15g
- Carbohydrates: 18g

- Fat: 10g
- Fiber: 3g
- Sugar: 12g
- Portion Size: 1 serving

Berry Blast Smoothie Bowl

Ingredients:

- 1 cup mixed berries (strawberries, blueberries, raspberries)
- 1/2 banana, frozen
- 1/2 cup unsweetened almond milk
- 1 tablespoon chia seeds
- 1 tablespoon almond butter
- Granola for topping (optional)

Instructions:

1. Blend mixed berries, frozen banana, almond milk, chia seeds, and almond butter until smooth.
2. Pour into a bowl and top with granola if desired.
3. Enjoy this refreshing and nutrient-packed smoothie bowl.

Nutrition Information:

- Calories: 280
- Protein: 8g
- Carbohydrates: 35g
- Fat: 14g
- Fiber: 10g
- Sugar: 15g
- Portion Size: 1 bowl

Avocado and Turkey Wrap

Ingredients:

- 1 whole-grain wrap
- 1/4 avocado, sliced
- 3 ounces turkey breast, sliced
- 1/2 cup spinach leaves
- 1 tablespoon Greek yogurt (plain, unsweetened)
- Salt and pepper to taste

Instructions:

1. Lay the whole-grain wrap on a flat surface.
2. Spread Greek yogurt over the wrap.
3. Layer sliced avocado, turkey, and spinach.

4. Season with salt and pepper to taste.

5. Roll the wrap tightly and cut in half.

6. Serve and relish the nutritious goodness.

Nutrition Information:

- Calories: 320
- Protein: 22g
- Carbohydrates: 26g
- Fat: 15g
- Fiber: 8g
- Sugar: 2g
- Portion Size: 1 wrap

Quinoa Breakfast Casserole

Ingredients:

- 1 cup cooked quinoa
- 2 eggs
- 1/2 cup milk (almond or skim)
- 1 cup diced vegetables (bell peppers, onions, spinach)
- 1/2 cup shredded cheese (cheddar or feta)
- Salt and pepper to taste

Instructions:

1. Preheat the oven to 350°F (175°C).

2. In a bowl, whisk together eggs and milk.

3. Stir in cooked quinoa, diced vegetables, and shredded cheese.

4. Season with salt and pepper.

5. Transfer the mixture to a greased baking dish.

6. Bake for 25-30 minutes or until set.

7. Slice and serve warm.

Nutrition Information:

- Calories: 280
- Protein: 15g
- Carbohydrates: 22g
- Fat: 14g
- Fiber: 3g
- Sugar: 2g
- Portion Size: 1 serving

Spinach and Feta Scramble

Ingredients:

- 2 large eggs

- 1 cup fresh spinach, chopped
- 2 tablespoons crumbled feta cheese
- 1 tablespoon olive oil
- Salt and pepper to taste

Instructions:

1. In a pan, heat olive oil over medium heat.
2. Add chopped spinach and sauté until wilted.
3. Beat eggs and pour them over the spinach.
4. Stir gently until eggs are almost set.
5. Add crumbled feta, salt, and pepper.
6. Continue cooking until eggs are fully cooked.
7. Plate and enjoy this flavorful and protein-packed scramble.

Nutrition Information:

- Calories: 230
- Protein: 14g
- Carbohydrates: 4g
- Fat: 18g
- Fiber: 2g
- Sugar: 1g

- Portion Size: 1 serving

Whole Grain Pancakes with Berries

Ingredients:

- 1/2 cup whole wheat flour
- 1/2 cup almond milk (unsweetened)
- 1 egg
- 1 tablespoon Greek yogurt (plain)
- 1 teaspoon baking powder
- Mixed berries for topping

Instructions:

1. In a bowl, whisk together whole wheat flour, almond milk, egg, Greek yogurt, and baking powder.
2. Heat a non-stick pan over medium heat.
3. Pour batter onto the pan to form pancakes.
4. Cook until bubbles form, then flip and cook the other side.
5. Top with mixed berries and serve warm.

Nutrition Information:

- Calories: 260

- Protein: 10g

- Carbohydrates: 40g

- Fat: 6g

- Fiber: 6g

- Sugar: 6g

- Portion Size: 2 pancakes

Chia Seed Pudding

Ingredients:

- 2 tablespoons chia seeds

- 1/2 cup almond milk (unsweetened)

- 1/4 teaspoon vanilla extract

- 1 tablespoon sugar-free sweetener

- Fresh berries for topping

Instructions:

1. In a bowl, combine chia seeds, almond milk, vanilla extract, and sweetener.

2. Stir well and let it sit for at least 2 hours or overnight in the refrigerator.

3. Stir again before serving.

4. Top with fresh berries and enjoy this nutritious chia seed pudding.

Nutrition Information:

- Calories: 120
- Protein: 4g
- Carbohydrates: 14g
- Fat: 6g
- Fiber: 8g
- Sugar: 2g
- Portion Size: 1 serving

Apple Cinnamon Steel-Cut Oats

Ingredients:

- 1/2 cup steel-cut oats
- 1 cup water
- 1/2 apple, diced
- 1/2 teaspoon ground cinnamon
- 1 tablespoon chopped nuts (walnuts or almonds)
- 1 teaspoon honey (optional)

Instructions:

1. In a saucepan, bring water to a boil.
2. Add steel-cut oats, reduce heat, and simmer until oats are tender.
3. Stir in diced apple, cinnamon, and chopped nuts.
4. Cook for an additional 5 minutes.
5. Drizzle with honey if desired and serve warm.

Nutrition Information:

- Calories: 220
- Protein: 7g
- Carbohydrates: 38g
- Fat: 5g
- Fiber: 6g
- Sugar: 10g
- Portion Size: 1 serving

Smoked Salmon Bagel Stack

Ingredients:

- 1 whole-grain bagel, sliced
- 2 ounces smoked salmon
- 2 tablespoons cream cheese (light)

- Capers for garnish

- Fresh dill for garnish

Instructions:

1. Toast the whole-grain bagel slices.

2. Spread cream cheese on each bagel half.

3. Layer smoked salmon on top of the cream cheese.

4. Garnish with capers and fresh dill.

5. Assemble the bagel stack and enjoy this elegant breakfast.

Nutrition Information:

- Calories: 280

- Protein: 15g

- Carbohydrates: 35g

- Fat: 10g

- Fiber: 4g

- Sugar: 2g

- Portion Size: 1 bagel stack

Sweet Potato Hash with Eggs

Ingredients:

- 1 medium sweet potato, grated
- 2 eggs
- 1/4 cup diced bell peppers
- 1/4 cup diced onions
- 1 tablespoon olive oil
- Salt and pepper to taste

Instructions:

1. In a skillet, heat olive oil over medium heat.
2. Add grated sweet potato, bell peppers, and onions.
3. Sauté until sweet potato is tender and lightly browned.
4. Create wells in the hash and crack eggs into them.
5. Cover and cook until eggs are done to your liking.
6. Season with salt and pepper.
7. Serve warm and enjoy this hearty breakfast.

Nutrition Information:

- Calories: 320
- Protein: 12g

- Carbohydrates: 30g

- Fat: 18g

- Fiber: 6g

- Sugar: 8g

- Portion Size: 1 serving

Cottage Cheese and Fruit Bowl

Ingredients:

- 1/2 cup low-fat cottage cheese

- 1/2 cup mixed fresh fruit (berries, melon, grapes)

- 1 tablespoon chopped nuts (almonds or walnuts)

- 1 teaspoon honey (optional)

Instructions:

1. In a bowl, place the low-fat cottage cheese.

2. Top with mixed fresh fruit and chopped nuts.

3. Drizzle with honey for added sweetness if desired.

4. Gently mix and enjoy this simple yet satisfying fruit bowl.

Nutrition Information:

- Calories: 200

- Protein: 15g

- Carbohydrates: 20g

- Fat: 8g

- Fiber: 3g

- Sugar: 15g

- Portion Size: 1 serving

Almond Butter Banana Toast

Ingredients:

- 1 slice whole-grain bread

- 1 tablespoon almond butter

- 1/2 banana, sliced

- 1 teaspoon chia seeds

- Cinnamon for sprinkling

Instructions:

1. Toast the whole-grain bread slice.

2. Spread almond butter over the toast.

3. Arrange banana slices on top.

4. Sprinkle chia seeds and cinnamon for extra flavor.

5. Enjoy this quick and tasty almond butter banana toast.

Nutrition Information:

- Calories: 230
- Protein: 6g
- Carbohydrates: 30g
- Fat: 10g
- Fiber: 6g
- Sugar: 10g
- Portion Size: 1 serving

Veggie Breakfast Burrito

Ingredients:

- 1 whole-grain tortilla
- 2 large eggs, scrambled
- 1/4 cup black beans, drained and rinsed
- 1/4 cup diced tomatoes
- 2 tablespoons diced onions
- 1/4 avocado, sliced
- Salsa for topping
- Fresh cilantro for garnish

Instructions:

1. In a pan, scramble the eggs until cooked through.

2. Warm the whole-grain tortilla.

3. Assemble the burrito by placing scrambled eggs in the center.

4. Add black beans, diced tomatoes, diced onions, and avocado slices.

5. Top with salsa and garnish with fresh cilantro.

6. Roll up the tortilla and enjoy this savory breakfast burrito.

Nutrition Information:

- Calories: 330
- Protein: 18g
- Carbohydrates: 35g
- Fat: 14g
- Fiber: 8g
- Sugar: 3g
- Portion Size: 1 burrito

Chapter 3: Lunch Recipes

In this chapter, we delve into a variety of tantalizing lunch recipes that not only cater to the palate but also adhere to a diabetic-friendly diet. Packed with wholesome ingredients and vibrant flavors, these lunch options aim to make your midday meal not just a necessity but a delightful experience.

Grilled Chicken Salad with Lemon Vinaigrette

Ingredients:

- 1 lb boneless, skinless chicken breasts
- 6 cups mixed salad greens
- 1 cup cherry tomatoes, halved
- 1 cucumber, sliced
- 1/4 cup feta cheese, crumbled
- 1/4 cup black olives, sliced

Lemon Vinaigrette:

- 3 tbsp olive oil
- 2 tbsp lemon juice

- 1 tsp Dijon mustard
- Salt and pepper to taste

Instructions:

1. Grill chicken until fully cooked, then slice.
2. In a large bowl, combine salad greens, cherry tomatoes, cucumber, feta, and olives.
3. Whisk together vinaigrette ingredients and drizzle over the salad.
4. Top the salad with grilled chicken slices.

Nutrition Information (per serving):

- Calories: 350
- Protein: 30g
- Carbohydrates: 15g
- Fat: 20g
- Fiber: 5g
- Sugar: 4g
- Portion Size: 1 serving

Quinoa and Black Bean Stuffed Peppers

Ingredients:

- 4 bell peppers, halved
- 1 cup cooked quinoa
- 1 can black beans, drained and rinsed
- 1 cup corn kernels
- 1 cup diced tomatoes
- 1 tsp cumin
- 1 tsp chili powder
- Salt and pepper to taste

Instructions:

1. Preheat the oven to 375°F (190°C).
2. In a bowl, mix quinoa, black beans, corn, diced tomatoes, cumin, chili powder, salt, and pepper.
3. Stuff the bell peppers with the quinoa mixture.
4. Bake for 25-30 minutes or until peppers are tender.

Nutrition Information (per serving):

- Calories: 280
- Protein: 12g

- Carbohydrates: 50g

- Fat: 3g

- Fiber: 10g

- Sugar: 8g

- Portion Size: 2 halves

Turkey and Avocado Wrap

Ingredients:

- 4 whole wheat wraps

- 1 lb turkey breast, sliced

- 2 avocados, sliced

- 1 cup lettuce, shredded

- 1/2 cup cherry tomatoes, halved

- 1/4 cup Greek yogurt

- Salt and pepper to taste

Instructions:

1. Lay out the wraps and evenly distribute turkey, avocado, lettuce, and cherry tomatoes on each.

2. Drizzle Greek yogurt over the fillings and season with salt and pepper.

3. Wrap tightly and slice in half.

Nutrition Information (per serving):

- Calories: 420
- Protein: 30g
- Carbohydrates: 45g
- Fat: 15g
- Fiber: 8g
- Sugar: 4g
- Portion Size: 1 wrap

Lentil and Vegetable Soup

Ingredients:

- 1 cup dried lentils, rinsed
- 1 onion, diced
- 2 carrots, sliced
- 2 celery stalks, chopped
- 3 cloves garlic, minced
- 1 can diced tomatoes
- 6 cups vegetable broth
- 1 tsp cumin
- 1 tsp paprika
- Salt and pepper to taste

Instructions:

1. In a large pot, sauté onions, carrots, celery, and garlic until softened.

2. Add lentils, diced tomatoes, vegetable broth, cumin, paprika, salt, and pepper.

3. Bring to a boil, then simmer for 25-30 minutes.

Nutrition Information (per serving):

- Calories: 250
- Protein: 15g
- Carbohydrates: 40g
- Fat: 2g
- Fiber: 15g
- Sugar: 5g
- Portion Size: 1.5 cups

Shrimp and Quinoa Bowl

Ingredients:

- 1 lb shrimp, peeled and deveined
- 2 cups cooked quinoa
- 1 cup broccoli florets
- 1 bell pepper, sliced

- 1/4 cup soy sauce
- 2 tbsp sesame oil
- 1 tbsp honey
- 1 tsp ginger, grated
- Sesame seeds for garnish

Instructions:

1. In a pan, cook shrimp until pink and opaque.
2. Steam broccoli until tender-crisp.
3. In a bowl, combine cooked quinoa, shrimp, broccoli, and bell pepper.
4. In a small bowl, whisk together soy sauce, sesame oil, honey, and ginger. Pour over the bowl and toss.
5. Garnish with sesame seeds.

Nutrition Information (per serving):

- Calories: 320
- Protein: 25g
- Carbohydrates: 35g
- Fat: 10g
- Fiber: 5g
- Sugar: 8g

- Portion Size: 1.5 cups

Caprese Salad with Balsamic Glaze

Ingredients:

- 4 large tomatoes, sliced
- 1 lb fresh mozzarella, sliced
- 1/2 cup fresh basil leaves
- 2 tbsp balsamic glaze
- Salt and pepper to taste

Instructions:

1. Arrange tomato and mozzarella slices on a serving platter, alternating with fresh basil leaves.
2. Drizzle balsamic glaze over the salad.
3. Season with salt and pepper.

Nutrition Information (per serving):

- Calories: 280
- Protein: 18g
- Carbohydrates: 10g
- Fat: 20g
- Fiber: 2g

- Sugar: 6g
- Portion Size: 1 plate

Chickpea and Vegetable Stir-Fry

Ingredients:

- 2 cups cooked chickpeas
- 1 cup broccoli florets
- 1 bell pepper, sliced
- 1 carrot, julienned
- 2 tbsp soy sauce
- 1 tbsp sesame oil
- 1 tsp garlic, minced
- 1 tsp ginger, grated

Instructions:

1. In a wok or skillet, stir-fry broccoli, bell pepper, and carrot until crisp-tender.
2. Add chickpeas, soy sauce, sesame oil, garlic, and ginger. Stir-fry for an additional 2-3 minutes.

Nutrition Information (per serving):

- Calories: 320

- Protein: 15g

- Carbohydrates: 45g

- Fat: 10g

- Fiber: 12g

- Sugar: 8g

- Portion Size: 1.5 cups

Salmon and Asparagus Foil Pack

Ingredients:

- 4 salmon fillets

- 1 bunch asparagus, trimmed

- 2 tbsp olive oil

- 2 tbsp lemon juice

- 2 cloves garlic, minced

- 1 tsp dill

- Salt and pepper to taste

Instructions:

1. Preheat the oven to 400°F (200°C).

2. Place each salmon fillet on a piece of foil. Arrange asparagus around the salmon.

3. In a bowl, whisk together olive oil, lemon juice, garlic, dill, salt, and pepper. Drizzle over salmon and asparagus.

4. Seal the foil packs and bake for 20 minutes.

Nutrition Information (per serving):

- Calories: 380
- Protein: 35g
- Carbohydrates: 10g
- Fat: 22g
- Fiber: 4g
- Sugar: 2g
- Portion Size: 1 foil pack

Zucchini Noodles with Pesto

Ingredients:

- 4 medium-sized zucchini, spiralized
- 1 cup cherry tomatoes, halved
- 1/2 cup pine nuts
- 1 cup fresh basil leaves
- 2 cloves garlic
- 1/2 cup grated Parmesan cheese

- 1/2 cup olive oil
- Salt and pepper to taste

Instructions:

1. In a blender or food processor, combine basil, pine nuts, garlic, and Parmesan. Blend until smooth.
2. With the blender running, slowly add olive oil until the pesto is well combined.
3. In a pan, sauté zucchini noodles until just tender.
4. Toss zucchini noodles with cherry tomatoes and pesto sauce.

Nutrition Information (per serving):

- Calories: 320
- Protein: 10g
- Carbohydrates: 12g
- Fat: 28g
- Fiber: 4g
- Sugar: 6g
- Portion Size: 2 cups

Greek Chicken Pita

Ingredients:

- 1 lb boneless, skinless chicken thighs
- 4 whole wheat pitas
- 1 cup Greek yogurt
- 1 cucumber, diced
- 1/2 cup cherry tomatoes, halved
- 1/4 cup red onion, finely chopped
- 1 tsp dried oregano
- Salt and pepper to taste

Instructions:

1. Grill chicken thighs until fully cooked.
2. In a bowl, combine Greek yogurt, cucumber, cherry tomatoes, red onion, oregano, salt, and pepper.
3. Slice the grilled chicken and stuff into whole wheat pitas. Top with the Greek yogurt mixture.

Nutrition Information (per serving):

- Calories: 380
- Protein: 30g
- Carbohydrates: 35g

- Fat: 15g
- Fiber: 5g
- Sugar: 6g
- Portion Size: 1 pita

Cauliflower Fried Rice

Ingredients:

- 4 cups cauliflower rice
- 1 cup mixed vegetables (peas, carrots, corn)
- 1 cup cooked shrimp, chopped
- 2 eggs, beaten
- 3 tbsp soy sauce
- 1 tbsp sesame oil
- 1 tsp ginger, minced
- 2 green onions, sliced

Instructions:

1. In a large pan, sauté cauliflower rice and mixed vegetables until tender.
2. Push the rice mixture to the side, pour beaten eggs into the pan, and scramble.

3. Add chopped shrimp, soy sauce, sesame oil, ginger,
   and green onions. Stir-fry until heated through.

Nutrition Information (per serving):

- Calories: 300
- Protein: 20g
- Carbohydrates: 20g
- Fat: 15g
- Fiber: 8g
- Sugar: 5g
- Portion Size: 1.5 cups

Tuna Salad Lettuce Wraps

Ingredients:

- 2 cans tuna, drained
- 1/2 cup celery, finely chopped
- 1/4 cup red onion, finely chopped
- 1/4 cup Greek yogurt
- 1 tbsp Dijon mustard
- Salt and pepper to taste
- Lettuce leaves for wrapping

Instructions:

1. In a bowl, mix tuna, celery, red onion, Greek yogurt, Dijon mustard, salt, and pepper.
2. Spoon the tuna salad onto lettuce leaves and wrap.

Nutrition Information (per serving):

- Calories: 220
- Protein: 25g
- Carbohydrates: 5g
- Fat: 10g
- Fiber: 2g
- Sugar: 2g
- Portion Size: 2 wraps

Turkey and Vegetable Skewers

Ingredients:

- 1 lb turkey breast, cut into cubes
- 1 zucchini, sliced
- 1 bell pepper, cut into chunks
- 1 red onion, cut into wedges
- 2 tbsp olive oil
- 1 tsp dried thyme

- Salt and pepper to taste

Instructions:

1. Preheat the grill.
2. Thread turkey cubes, zucchini slices, bell pepper chunks, and red onion wedges onto skewers.
3. In a bowl, mix olive oil, dried thyme, salt, and pepper. Brush over skewers.
4. Grill until turkey is cooked through and vegetables are tender.

Nutrition Information (per serving):

- Calories: 280
- Protein: 30g
- Carbohydrates: 10g
- Fat: 12g
- Fiber: 3g
- Sugar: 5g
- Portion Size: 2 skewers

Spinach and Mushroom Quesadilla

Ingredients:

- 4 whole wheat tortillas
- 2 cups spinach, chopped
- 1 cup mushrooms, sliced
- 1 cup shredded mozzarella cheese
- 1/4 cup red onion, thinly sliced
- 1 tsp olive oil
- 1 tsp cumin
- Salt and pepper to taste

Instructions:

1. In a pan, sauté spinach, mushrooms, and red onion in olive oil until wilted.
2. Place a tortilla in the pan, top with sautéed mixture and mozzarella. Place another tortilla on top.
3. Cook until cheese is melted and tortilla is golden brown, then flip and cook the other side.

Nutrition Information (per serving):

- Calories: 330
- Protein: 20g

- Carbohydrates: 30g

- Fat: 15g

- Fiber: 5g

- Sugar: 3g

- Portion Size: 1 quesadilla

Broccoli and Cheddar Stuffed Chicken Breast

Ingredients:

- 4 boneless, skinless chicken breasts

- 2 cups broccoli florets, steamed

- 1 cup cheddar cheese, shredded

- 1/4 cup plain Greek yogurt

- 2 cloves garlic, minced

- 1 tsp onion powder

- Salt and pepper to taste

Instructions:

1. Preheat the oven to 375°F (190°C).

2. Butterfly each chicken breast and season with salt and pepper.

3. In a bowl, mix steamed broccoli, cheddar cheese, Greek yogurt, garlic, and onion powder.

4. Stuff each chicken breast with the broccoli and cheddar mixture.

5. Bake for 25-30 minutes or until chicken is cooked through.

Nutrition Information (per serving):

- Calories: 340
- Protein: 40g
- Carbohydrates: 10g
- Fat: 15g
- Fiber: 3g
- Sugar: 2g
- Portion Size: 1 stuffed chicken breast

Chapter 4: Dinner Recipes

In this chapter, we've curated delightful dinner recipes that not only cater to your nutritional needs but also tantalize your taste buds. From succulent seafood to hearty vegetarian options, each recipe is thoughtfully crafted to ensure a satisfying and health-conscious dining experience.

Baked Cod with Lemon and Herbs:

Ingredients:

- 4 cod fillets
- 1 lemon (juiced and zested)
- 2 tablespoons olive oil
- 1 teaspoon dried oregano
- Salt and pepper to taste

Instructions:

1. Preheat the oven to 375°F (190°C).
2. Place cod fillets in a baking dish.
3. Mix lemon juice, zest, olive oil, oregano, salt, and pepper.

4. Pour the mixture over the cod.

5. Bake for 20-25 minutes or until the fish flakes easily.

Nutrition Information (per serving):

- Calories: 250

- Protein: 30g

- Carbohydrates: 3g

- Fat: 12g

- Fiber: 1g

- Sugar: 0g

- Portion Size: 1 fillet

Eggplant Lasagna:

Ingredients:

- 1 large eggplant

- 2 cups marinara sauce (sugar-free)

- 1 cup ricotta cheese (part-skim)

- 1 cup mozzarella cheese (part-skim, shredded)

- 1/2 cup Parmesan cheese (grated)

- 1 teaspoon dried basil

- Salt and pepper to taste

Instructions:

1. Preheat oven to 375°F (190°C).
2. Slice eggplant into thin rounds.
3. Layer eggplant, marinara sauce, ricotta, mozzarella, and Parmesan.
4. Repeat layers and sprinkle basil, salt, and pepper.
5. Bake for 30-35 minutes or until bubbly and golden.

Nutrition Information (per serving):

- Calories: 280
- Protein: 15g
- Carbohydrates: 15g
- Fat: 18g
- Fiber: 5g
- Sugar: 8g
- Portion Size: 1/6 of the lasagna

Cilantro Lime Chicken:

Ingredients:

- 4 boneless, skinless chicken breasts
- 1/4 cup fresh cilantro (chopped)
- 2 limes (juiced)

- 2 tablespoons olive oil

- 1 teaspoon cumin

- Salt and pepper to taste

Instructions:

1. Preheat grill or skillet over medium-high heat.

2. In a bowl, mix cilantro, lime juice, olive oil, cumin, salt, and pepper.

3. Coat chicken with the mixture and grill for 6-8 minutes per side.

Nutrition Information (per serving):

- Calories: 220

- Protein: 30g

- Carbohydrates: 2g

- Fat: 10g

- Fiber: 0g

- Sugar: 0g

- Portion Size: 1 chicken breast

Quinoa and Spinach Stuffed Mushrooms:

Ingredients:

- 12 large mushrooms (cleaned and stems removed)
- 1 cup cooked quinoa
- 1 cup fresh spinach (chopped)
- 1/2 cup feta cheese (crumbled)
- 2 cloves garlic (minced)
- Salt and pepper to taste

Instructions:

1. Preheat the oven to 375°F (190°C).
2. In a bowl, combine quinoa, spinach, feta, garlic, salt, and pepper.
3. Stuff mushrooms with the mixture and bake for 15-20 minutes.

Nutrition Information (per serving):

- Calories: 120
- Protein: 6g
- Carbohydrates: 15g
- Fat: 5g

- Fiber: 3g

- Sugar: 2g

- Portion Size: 4 stuffed mushrooms

Turkey and Sweet Potato Skillet:

Ingredients:

- 1 lb ground turkey

- 2 sweet potatoes (peeled and diced)

- 1 onion (chopped)

- 2 bell peppers (sliced)

- 1 tablespoon olive oil

- 1 teaspoon smoked paprika

- Salt and pepper to taste

Instructions:

1. In a large skillet, brown turkey in olive oil.

2. Add sweet potatoes, onion, and bell peppers. Cook until vegetables are tender.

3. Season with smoked paprika, salt, and pepper.

Nutrition Information (per serving):

- Calories: 300

- Protein: 20g

- Carbohydrates: 25g

- Fat: 12g

- Fiber: 5g

- Sugar: 7g

- Portion Size: 1 cup

Lemon Garlic Shrimp with Zoodles:

Ingredients:

- 1 lb shrimp (peeled and deveined)

- 3 zucchinis (spiralized into noodles)

- 3 cloves garlic (minced)

- 2 tablespoons olive oil

- 1 lemon (juiced)

- 1 teaspoon red pepper flakes

- Salt and pepper to taste

Instructions:

1. In a pan, sauté shrimp and garlic in olive oil until shrimp turn pink.

2. Add zoodles, lemon juice, red pepper flakes, salt, and pepper. Cook for 3-4 minutes.

Nutrition Information (per serving):

- Calories: 220
- Protein: 25g
- Carbohydrates: 10g
- Fat: 10g
- Fiber: 3g
- Sugar: 5g
- Portion Size: 1 cup

Asian-Inspired Salmon:

Ingredients:

- 4 salmon fillets
- 1/4 cup soy sauce (low-sodium)
- 2 tablespoons rice vinegar
- 1 tablespoon honey
- 1 teaspoon sesame oil
- 2 green onions (sliced)
- 1 teaspoon sesame seeds (for garnish)

Instructions:

1. Preheat oven to 400°F (200°C).

2. In a bowl, mix soy sauce, rice vinegar, honey, and sesame oil.

3. Place salmon fillets in a baking dish, pour the sauce over them, and bake for 15-20 minutes.

4. Garnish with green onions and sesame seeds.

Nutrition Information (per serving):

- Calories: 280
- Protein: 25g
- Carbohydrates: 8g
- Fat: 15g
- Fiber: 1g
- Sugar: 5g
- Portion Size: 1 fillet

Cauliflower and Chickpea Curry:

Ingredients:

- 1 cauliflower head (cut into florets)
- 1 can chickpeas (drained and rinsed)
- 1 onion (chopped)
- 2 tomatoes (chopped)
- 3 cloves garlic (minced)

- 1 tablespoon curry powder

- 1 teaspoon turmeric

- 1 cup vegetable broth

- Salt and pepper to taste

Instructions:

1. In a pot, sauté onions and garlic until softened.

2. Add cauliflower, chickpeas, tomatoes, curry powder, turmeric, and vegetable broth.

3. Simmer until cauliflower is tender.

Nutrition Information (per serving):

- Calories: 220

- Protein: 8g

- Carbohydrates: 40g

- Fat: 4g

- Fiber: 12g

- Sugar: 10g

- Portion Size: 1 cup

Grilled Vegetable Medley:

Ingredients:

- 2 zucchinis (sliced)
- 1 eggplant (sliced)
- 1 red bell pepper (sliced)
- 1 yellow bell pepper (sliced)
- 1 red onion (sliced)
- 2 tablespoons olive oil
- 1 teaspoon Italian seasoning
- Salt and pepper to taste

Instructions:

1. Preheat grill to medium-high heat.
2. Toss vegetables with olive oil, Italian seasoning, salt, and pepper.
3. Grill until tender and slightly charred.

Nutrition Information (per serving):

- Calories: 180
- Protein: 4g
- Carbohydrates: 20g
- Fat: 10g

- Fiber: 8g

- Sugar: 10g

- Portion Size: 1 cup

Balsamic Glazed Chicken Thighs:

Ingredients:

- 4 bone-in, skinless chicken thighs

- 1/4 cup balsamic vinegar

- 2 tablespoons olive oil

- 2 tablespoons honey

- 2 cloves garlic (minced)

- 1 teaspoon dried thyme

- Salt and pepper to taste

Instructions:

1. Preheat oven to 400°F (200°C).

2. In a bowl, mix balsamic vinegar, olive oil, honey, garlic, thyme, salt, and pepper.

3. Coat chicken thighs with the mixture and bake for 25-30 minutes.

Nutrition Information (per serving):

- Calories: 320

- Protein: 22g

- Carbohydrates: 10g

- Fat: 20g

- Fiber: 0g

- Sugar: 8g

- Portion Size: 1 thigh

Zesty Lemon Dill Tilapia:

Ingredients:

- 4 tilapia fillets

- 1 lemon (juiced and zested)

- 2 tablespoons fresh dill (chopped)

- 2 tablespoons olive oil

- 1 teaspoon garlic powder

- Salt and pepper to taste

Instructions:

1. Preheat oven to 375°F (190°C).

2. Place tilapia fillets in a baking dish.

3. Mix lemon juice, zest, dill, olive oil, garlic powder, salt, and pepper.

4. Pour the mixture over the tilapia and bake for 15-20 minutes.

Nutrition Information (per serving):

- Calories: 180
- Protein: 22g
- Carbohydrates: 2g
- Fat: 10g
- Fiber: 0g
- Sugar: 0g
- Portion Size: 1 fillet

Ratatouille with Brown Rice:

Ingredients:

- 1 eggplant (cubed)
- 2 zucchinis (sliced)
- 1 bell pepper (sliced)
- 1 onion (sliced)
- 2 tomatoes (chopped)
- 3 cloves garlic (minced)

- 2 tablespoons olive oil
- 1 teaspoon dried thyme
- Salt and pepper to taste
- 2 cups cooked brown rice

Instructions:

1. In a large pan, sauté onion and garlic in olive oil until softened.
2. Add eggplant, zucchini, bell pepper, tomatoes, thyme, salt, and pepper. Cook until vegetables are tender.
3. Serve over cooked brown rice.

Nutrition Information (per serving):

- Calories: 250
- Protein: 6g
- Carbohydrates: 40g
- Fat: 8g
- Fiber: 8g
- Sugar: 8g
- Portion Size: 1 cup

Turkey Chili:

Ingredients:

- 1 lb ground turkey
- 1 can kidney beans (drained and rinsed)
- 1 can diced tomatoes (low-sodium)
- 1 onion (chopped)
- 2 cloves garlic (minced)
- 1 tablespoon chili powder
- 1 teaspoon cumin
- Salt and pepper to taste

Instructions:

1. In a pot, brown turkey with onions and garlic.
2. Add beans, diced tomatoes, chili powder, cumin, salt, and pepper.
3. Simmer for 20-25 minutes.

Nutrition Information (per serving):

- Calories: 280
- Protein: 20g
- Carbohydrates: 25g
- Fat: 12g

- Fiber: 8g

- Sugar: 5g

- Portion Size: 1 cup

Spaghetti Squash Primavera:

Ingredients:

- 1 medium spaghetti squash

- 1 cup cherry tomatoes (halved)

- 1 cup broccoli florets

- 1 bell pepper (sliced)

- 2 tablespoons olive oil

- 2 cloves garlic (minced)

- 1 teaspoon Italian seasoning

- Salt and pepper to taste

Instructions:

1. Preheat oven to 400°F (200°C).

2. Cut spaghetti squash in half, scoop out seeds, and bake for 40-45 minutes.

3. In a pan, sauté garlic, add tomatoes, broccoli, bell pepper, Italian seasoning, salt, and pepper.

4. Scrape cooked squash into strands and toss with the vegetable mixture.

Nutrition Information (per serving):

- Calories: 180
- Protein: 4g
- Carbohydrates: 25g
- Fat: 8g
- Fiber: 6g
- Sugar: 10g
- Portion Size: 1 cup

Mexican Cauliflower Rice Bowl:

Ingredients:

- 1 head cauliflower (riced)
- 1 lb lean ground beef
- 1 cup black beans (canned, drained, and rinsed)
- 1 cup corn kernels (fresh or frozen)
- 1 cup salsa
- 1 teaspoon cumin
- 1 teaspoon chili powder
- Salt and pepper to taste

- Fresh cilantro for garnish

Instructions:

1. In a pan, brown ground beef, add cauliflower rice, black beans, corn, salsa, cumin, chili powder, salt, and pepper.
2. Cook until cauliflower is tender.
3. Garnish with fresh cilantro.

Nutrition Information (per serving):

- Calories: 320
- Protein: 25g
- Carbohydrates: 30g
- Fat: 12g
- Fiber: 10g
- Sugar: 5g
- Portion Size: 1 cup

Chapter 5: Snacks and Appetizers

These recipes are crafted to satisfy your cravings without compromising your health. Each bite is a burst of flavor and nutrition, ensuring a delightful snacking experience.

Hummus and Veggie Sticks

Ingredients:

- 1 cup chickpeas (canned, drained)
- 2 tablespoons tahini
- 2 tablespoons olive oil
- 1 clove garlic, minced
- 1 tablespoon lemon juice
- Assorted fresh vegetables (carrot sticks, cucumber, bell pepper) for dipping

Instructions:

1. In a food processor, combine chickpeas, tahini, olive oil, garlic, and lemon juice.
2. Blend until smooth and creamy.
3. Serve with fresh veggie sticks.

Nutrition Information (per serving):

- Calories: 120
- Protein: 4g
- Carbohydrates: 15g
- Fat: 6g
- Fiber: 4g
- Sugar: 2g
- Portion Size: 2 tablespoons hummus with veggies

Cheese and Grape Skewers

Ingredients:

- Cubes of low-fat cheese (cheddar, mozzarella)
- Red and green grapes

Instructions:

1. Thread a grape followed by a cheese cube onto a toothpick or skewer.
2. Repeat the process for each skewer.
3. Arrange on a platter and serve.

Nutrition Information (per serving):

- Calories: 80

- Protein: 5g

- Carbohydrates: 10g

- Fat: 4g

- Fiber: 1g

- Sugar: 7g

- Portion Size: 4 skewers

Cucumber and Cream Cheese Bites

Ingredients:

- Cucumber slices

- Low-fat cream cheese

- Fresh dill, chopped

Instructions:

1. Spread a thin layer of cream cheese on each cucumber slice.

2. Sprinkle with chopped dill.

3. Arrange on a serving platter and enjoy.

Nutrition Information (per serving):

- Calories: 50

- Protein: 2g

- Carbohydrates: 3g
- Fat: 3g
- Fiber: 1g
- Sugar: 2g
- Portion Size: 5 pieces

Edamame with Sea Salt

Ingredients:

- Edamame beans (shelled)
- Sea salt

Instructions:

1. Steam edamame beans until tender.
2. Sprinkle with sea salt and toss to coat.
3. Serve in a bowl and enjoy this protein-packed snack.

Nutrition Information (per serving):

- Calories: 90
- Protein: 8g
- Carbohydrates: 8g
- Fat: 3g
- Fiber: 4g

- Sugar: 2g
- Portion Size: 1 cup

Almond and Cranberry Energy Bites

Ingredients:

- 1 cup almonds, finely chopped
- 1/2 cup dried cranberries, chopped
- 2 tablespoons almond butter
- 1 tablespoon honey
- 1/2 teaspoon vanilla extract

Instructions:

1. In a bowl, combine almonds, cranberries, almond butter, honey, and vanilla extract.
2. Mix until well combined.
3. Form into bite-sized balls and refrigerate for at least 30 minutes.

Nutrition Information (per serving):

- Calories: 100
- Protein: 3g
- Carbohydrates: 10g

- Fat: 6g
- Fiber: 2g
- Sugar: 6g
- Portion Size: 2 energy bites

Avocado Salsa with Whole Grain Chips

Ingredients:

- 2 ripe avocados, diced
- 1 cup tomatoes, diced
- 1/4 cup red onion, finely chopped
- 1/4 cup fresh cilantro, chopped
- 1 lime, juiced
- Salt and pepper to taste
- Whole grain tortilla chips

Instructions:

1. In a bowl, combine avocados, tomatoes, red onion, cilantro, and lime juice.
2. Season with salt and pepper to taste.
3. Serve with whole grain tortilla chips.

Nutrition Information (per serving):

- Calories: 120
- Protein: 2g
- Carbohydrates: 15g
- Fat: 7g
- Fiber: 5g
- Sugar: 2g
- Portion Size: 1/2 cup salsa with chips

Greek Yogurt and Berries Parfait

Ingredients:

- 1 cup Greek yogurt
- Mixed berries (strawberries, blueberries, raspberries)
- 1 tablespoon honey
- Granola (optional)

Instructions:

1. In a glass, layer Greek yogurt, mixed berries, and honey.
2. Repeat the layers until the glass is filled.
3. Top with granola if desired and serve.

Nutrition Information (per serving):

- Calories: 150
- Protein: 10g
- Carbohydrates: 20g
- Fat: 3g
- Fiber: 4g
- Sugar: 12g
- Portion Size: 1 parfait

Roasted Red Pepper and Feta Dip

Ingredients:

- 1 cup roasted red peppers, drained and chopped
- 1/2 cup feta cheese, crumbled
- 2 tablespoons Greek yogurt
- 1 clove garlic, minced
- 1 tablespoon olive oil
- Fresh herbs for garnish

Instructions:

1. In a food processor, combine roasted red peppers, feta cheese, Greek yogurt, garlic, and olive oil.
2. Blend until smooth and creamy.

3. Garnish with fresh herbs and serve with vegetable sticks or whole grain crackers.

Nutrition Information (per serving):

- Calories: 90
- Protein: 4g
- Carbohydrates: 5g
- Fat: 6g
- Fiber: 1g
- Sugar: 3g
- Portion Size: 2 tablespoons dip

Apple Slices with Peanut Butter

Ingredients:

- Apple slices
- Natural peanut butter

Instructions:

1. Spread peanut butter on apple slices.
2. Arrange on a plate and enjoy this simple and satisfying snack.

Nutrition Information (per serving):

- Calories: 120
- Protein: 3g
- Carbohydrates: 15g
- Fat: 7g
- Fiber: 3g
- Sugar: 9g
- Portion Size: 1 apple with 2 tablespoons peanut butter

Caprese Kabobs

Ingredients:

- Cherry tomatoes
- Fresh mozzarella balls
- Basil leaves
- Balsamic glaze for drizzling

Instructions:

1. Thread a tomato, mozzarella ball, and basil leaf onto toothpicks.
2. Arrange on a serving platter and drizzle with balsamic glaze.

Nutrition Information (per serving):

- Calories: 70
- Protein: 4g
- Carbohydrates: 2g
- Fat: 5g
- Fiber: 1g
- Sugar: 1g
- Portion Size: 4 kabobs

Spicy Roasted Chickpeas

Ingredients:

- 1 can chickpeas, drained and rinsed
- 1 tablespoon olive oil
- 1 teaspoon paprika
- 1/2 teaspoon cayenne pepper
- Salt and pepper to taste

Instructions:

1. Preheat the oven to 400°F (200°C).
2. In a bowl, toss chickpeas with olive oil, paprika, cayenne pepper, salt, and pepper.

3. Spread on a baking sheet and roast for 20-25 minutes until crispy.

Nutrition Information (per serving):

- Calories: 100
- Protein: 4g
- Carbohydrates: 15g
- Fat: 3g
- Fiber: 4g
- Sugar: 3g
- Portion Size: 1/2 cup

Nut Mix with Dried Fruit

Ingredients:

- 1/2 cup mixed nuts (almonds, walnuts, pistachios)
- 1/4 cup dried fruits (apricots, cranberries, raisins)
- 1 teaspoon cinnamon

Instructions:

1. Combine mixed nuts and dried fruits in a bowl.
2. Sprinkle with cinnamon and toss to coat.

3. Serve in portioned cups for a satisfying and nutritious snack.

Nutrition Information (per serving):

- Calories: 120
- Protein: 4g
- Carbohydrates: 10g
- Fat: 8g
- Fiber: 2g
- Sugar: 5g
- Portion Size: 1/4 cup

Guacamole with Jicama Slices

Ingredients:

- 2 ripe avocados
- 1 tomato, diced
- 1/4 cup red onion, finely chopped
- 1 clove garlic, minced
- Lime juice to taste
- Salt and pepper to taste
- Jicama slices for dipping

Instructions:

1. Mash avocados in a bowl and add diced tomato, red onion, garlic, lime juice, salt, and pepper.
2. Mix until well combined.
3. Serve with jicama slices for a crunchy and refreshing dip.

Nutrition Information (per serving):

- Calories: 110
- Protein: 2g
- Carbohydrates: 8g
- Fat: 9g
- Fiber: 5g
- Sugar: 2g
- Portion Size: 1/2 cup guacamole with jicama slices

Cottage Cheese and Pineapple Cups

Ingredients:

- 1 cup low-fat cottage cheese
- 1 cup fresh pineapple chunks
- Mint leaves for garnish

Instructions:

1. In a bowl, combine cottage cheese and pineapple chunks.

2. Spoon into individual cups and garnish with mint leaves.

3. Enjoy this sweet and savory snack.

Nutrition Information (per serving):

- Calories: 140
- Protein: 15g
- Carbohydrates: 20g
- Fat: 2g
- Fiber: 2g
- Sugar: 15g
- Portion Size: 1 cup

Tomato Basil Bruschetta

Ingredients:

- 4 ripe tomatoes, diced
- 1/4 cup fresh basil, chopped
- 2 cloves garlic, minced
- 2 tablespoons balsamic vinegar

- 1 tablespoon olive oil
- Whole grain baguette slices for serving

Instructions:

1. In a bowl, combine tomatoes, basil, garlic, balsamic vinegar, and olive oil.
2. Mix well and let it marinate for 15 minutes.
3. Serve on whole grain baguette slices for a flavorful bruschetta.

Nutrition Information (per serving):

- Calories: 80
- Protein: 2g
- Carbohydrates: 12g
- Fat: 3g
- Fiber: 2g
- Sugar: 4g
- Portion Size: 2 tablespoons bruschetta on 2 slices of baguette

Chapter 6: Desserts

This chapter presents a delightful array of desserts specially crafted for beginners, ensuring that each treat is both scrumptious and mindful of your dietary needs. Let's dive into the sweetness without any guilt!

Sugar-Free Chocolate Avocado Mousse

Ingredients:

- 2 ripe avocados
- 1/2 cup unsweetened cocoa powder
- 1/4 cup almond milk
- 1/4 cup sugar substitute
- 1 teaspoon vanilla extract
- Pinch of salt

Instructions:

1. Peel and pit avocados, placing the flesh in a blender.
2. Add cocoa powder, almond milk, sugar substitute, vanilla extract, and a pinch of salt.

3. Blend until smooth and creamy.

4. Refrigerate for at least 2 hours before serving.

Nutrition Information (per serving):

- Calories: 150

- Protein: 3g

- Carbohydrates: 12g

- Fat: 11g

- Fiber: 7g

- Sugar: 1g

- Portion Size: 1/2 cup

Berry and Greek Yogurt Popsicles

Ingredients:

- 1 cup mixed berries (strawberries, blueberries, raspberries)

- 1 cup Greek yogurt (unsweetened)

- 2 tablespoons honey (optional)

Instructions:

1. Blend mixed berries until smooth.

2. In a separate bowl, mix Greek yogurt with honey.

3. Layer the berry puree and yogurt in popsicle molds.

4. Insert popsicle sticks and freeze for at least 4 hours.

Nutrition Information (per popsicle):

- Calories: 60

- Protein: 4g

- Carbohydrates: 10g

- Fat: 0.5g

- Fiber: 2g

- Sugar: 7g

- Portion Size: 1 popsicle

Almond Flour Pumpkin Muffins

Ingredients:

- 1 cup almond flour

- 1/2 cup canned pumpkin puree

- 1/4 cup coconut oil (melted)

- 1/4 cup sugar substitute

- 2 eggs

- 1 teaspoon baking powder

- 1/2 teaspoon cinnamon

- Pinch of salt

Instructions:

1. Preheat oven to 350°F (175°C) and line a muffin tin with paper liners.
2. In a bowl, mix almond flour, pumpkin puree, melted coconut oil, sugar substitute, eggs, baking powder, cinnamon, and a pinch of salt.
3. Spoon the batter into muffin cups and bake for 20-25 minutes.

Nutrition Information (per muffin):

- Calories: 120
- Protein: 5g
- Carbohydrates: 6g
- Fat: 10g
- Fiber: 3g
- Sugar: 1g
- Portion Size: 1 muffin

Dark Chocolate Covered Strawberries

Ingredients:

- 1 cup dark chocolate chips (sugar-free)
- 1 pint fresh strawberries, washed and dried

Instructions:

1. Melt dark chocolate chips in a microwave-safe bowl.
2. Dip each strawberry into the melted chocolate, covering them halfway.
3. Place on parchment paper and refrigerate until the chocolate hardens.

Nutrition Information (per serving, 2 strawberries):

- Calories: 90
- Protein: 1g
- Carbohydrates: 12g
- Fat: 5g
- Fiber: 3g
- Sugar: 6g
- Portion Size: 2 strawberries

Lemon Chia Seed Pudding

Ingredients:

- 1/4 cup chia seeds
- 1 cup almond milk
- Zest and juice of 1 lemon
- 2 tablespoons sugar substitute
- 1/2 teaspoon vanilla extract

Instructions:

1. In a bowl, mix chia seeds, almond milk, lemon zest, lemon juice, sugar substitute, and vanilla extract.
2. Refrigerate for at least 4 hours or overnight, stirring occasionally.

Nutrition Information (per serving):

- Calories: 80
- Protein: 3g
- Carbohydrates: 9g
- Fat: 4g
- Fiber: 6g
- Sugar: 1g
- Portion Size: 1/2 cup

Baked Apple with Cinnamon

Ingredients:

- 2 apples, cored and halved
- 1 teaspoon cinnamon
- 1 tablespoon sugar substitute
- 1 tablespoon chopped nuts (optional)

Instructions:

1. Preheat oven to 375°F (190°C).
2. Place apple halves in a baking dish, sprinkle with cinnamon and sugar substitute.
3. Bake for 25-30 minutes until apples are tender.
4. Garnish with chopped nuts if desired.

Nutrition Information (per serving, 1 apple half):

- Calories: 50
- Protein: 0.5g
- Carbohydrates: 12g
- Fat: 0.5g
- Fiber: 2g
- Sugar: 8g
- Portion Size: 1 apple half

Avocado Chocolate Pudding

Ingredients:

- 2 ripe avocados
- 1/4 cup unsweetened cocoa powder
- 1/4 cup almond milk
- 1/4 cup sugar substitute
- 1 teaspoon vanilla extract
- Pinch of salt

Instructions:

1. Scoop the avocados into a blender.
2. Add cocoa powder, almond milk, sugar substitute, vanilla extract, and a pinch of salt.
3. Blend until smooth and creamy.
4. Refrigerate for at least 2 hours before serving.

Nutrition Information (per serving):

- Calories: 140
- Protein: 2g
- Carbohydrates: 10g
- Fat: 11g
- Fiber: 6g

- Sugar: 1g
- Portion Size: 1/2 cup

Coconut Flour Blueberry Bars

Ingredients:

- 1 cup coconut flour
- 1/2 cup almond flour
- 1/4 cup coconut oil (melted)
- 1/4 cup sugar substitute
- 2 eggs
- 1 teaspoon vanilla extract
- 1/2 cup fresh blueberries

Instructions:

1. Preheat oven to 350°F (175°C) and grease a baking pan.
2. In a bowl, combine coconut flour, almond flour, melted coconut oil, sugar substitute, eggs, and vanilla extract.
3. Fold in the blueberries and spread the batter in the prepared pan.

4. Bake for 25-30 minutes until edges are golden brown.

Nutrition Information (per serving):

- Calories: 120
- Protein: 4g
- Carbohydrates: 8g
- Fat: 9g
- Fiber: 4g
- Sugar: 2g
- Portion Size: 1 bar

Pistachio and Cherry Frozen Yogurt

Ingredients:

- 2 cups Greek yogurt (unsweetened)
- 1/2 cup shelled pistachios, chopped
- 1/2 cup cherries, pitted and chopped
- 1/4 cup sugar substitute
- 1 teaspoon vanilla extract

Instructions:

1. In a bowl, mix Greek yogurt, chopped pistachios, chopped cherries, sugar substitute, and vanilla extract.
2. Transfer the mixture to an ice cream maker and churn according to the manufacturer's instructions.
3. Freeze for an additional 2 hours before serving.

Nutrition Information (per serving):

- Calories: 130
- Protein: 8g
- Carbohydrates: 10g
- Fat: 7g
- Fiber: 2g
- Sugar: 5g
- Portion Size: 1/2 cup

Raspberry Almond Tart

Ingredients:

- 1 cup almond flour
- 1/4 cup coconut oil (melted)
- 2 tablespoons sugar substitute

- 1 cup fresh raspberries
- 1/4 cup sugar-free raspberry jam
- Fresh mint leaves for garnish

Instructions:

1. Preheat oven to 350°F (175°C) and grease a tart pan.
2. In a bowl, combine almond flour, melted coconut oil, and sugar substitute.
3. Press the mixture into the tart pan to form the crust and bake for 12-15 minutes.
4. Allow the crust to cool, then spread sugar-free raspberry jam over it.
5. Arrange fresh raspberries on top and garnish with mint leaves.

Nutrition Information (per serving):

- Calories: 150
- Protein: 3g
- Carbohydrates: 8g
- Fat: 12g
- Fiber: 4g
- Sugar: 2g

- Portion Size: 1 slice

Vanilla Bean Panna Cotta

Ingredients:

- 1 cup heavy cream
- 1 cup unsweetened almond milk
- 1/4 cup sugar substitute
- 1 vanilla bean, split and seeds scraped
- 2 teaspoons gelatin
- Fresh berries for topping

Instructions:

1. In a saucepan, heat heavy cream, almond milk, sugar substitute, and vanilla bean seeds over medium heat.
2. Sprinkle gelatin over the mixture and whisk until dissolved.
3. Remove from heat, discard the vanilla bean, and pour into serving glasses.
4. Refrigerate for at least 4 hours or until set.
5. Top with fresh berries before serving.

Nutrition Information (per serving):

- Calories: 180
- Protein: 2g
- Carbohydrates: 5g
- Fat: 17g
- Fiber: 0g
- Sugar: 2g
- Portion Size: 1/2 cup

Mixed Berry Sorbet

Ingredients:

- 2 cups mixed berries (strawberries, blueberries, raspberries)
- 1/4 cup sugar substitute
- 1 tablespoon lemon juice
- 1/4 cup water

Instructions:

1. In a blender, combine mixed berries, sugar substitute, lemon juice, and water.
2. Blend until smooth and pour into a shallow dish.

3. Freeze for 2-3 hours, stirring every 30 minutes until
    sorbet reaches desired consistency.

Nutrition Information (per serving):

- Calories: 60
- Protein: 1g
- Carbohydrates: 15g
- Fat: 0.5g
- Fiber: 4g
- Sugar: 8g
- Portion Size: 1/2 cup

Pumpkin Pie Smoothie

Ingredients:

- 1/2 cup canned pumpkin puree
- 1 cup unsweetened almond milk
- 1/2 banana
- 1/2 teaspoon pumpkin spice
- 1 tablespoon chia seeds
- 1 tablespoon sugar substitute
- Ice cubes

Instructions:

1. In a blender, combine pumpkin puree, almond milk, banana, pumpkin spice, chia seeds, sugar substitute, and ice cubes.

2. Blend until smooth and creamy.

3. Pour into a glass and sprinkle a dash of pumpkin spice on top.

Nutrition Information (per serving):

- Calories: 120
- Protein: 3g
- Carbohydrates: 15g
- Fat: 6g
- Fiber: 6g
- Sugar: 4g
- Portion Size: 1 cup

Walnut and Date Energy Balls

Ingredients:

- 1 cup walnuts
- 1 cup dates, pitted
- 1 tablespoon cocoa powder

- 1 teaspoon vanilla extract
- Pinch of salt
- Unsweetened shredded coconut for coating

Instructions:

1. In a food processor, blend walnuts, dates, cocoa powder, vanilla extract, and a pinch of salt until the mixture forms a sticky dough.
2. Roll the dough into bite-sized balls and coat with shredded coconut.
3. Refrigerate for at least 1 hour before serving.

Nutrition Information (per serving, 2 energy balls):

- Calories: 100
- Protein: 2g
- Carbohydrates: 12g
- Fat: 6g
- Fiber: 2g
- Sugar: 8g
- Portion Size: 2 energy balls

Grilled Peaches with Honey Drizzle

Ingredients:

- 2 peaches, halved and pitted
- 1 tablespoon coconut oil (melted)
- 1 tablespoon honey (sugar-free)
- Cinnamon for sprinkling

Instructions:

1. Preheat the grill or grill pan.
2. Brush peach halves with melted coconut oil.
3. Grill for 2-3 minutes on each side until grill marks appear.
4. Drizzle with sugar-free honey and sprinkle with cinnamon before serving.

Nutrition Information (per serving, 2 peach halves):

- Calories: 90
- Protein: 1g
- Carbohydrates: 20g
- Fat: 3g
- Fiber: 3g
- Sugar: 17g
- Portion Size: 2 peach halves

Chapter 7: Smoothies

These refreshing concoctions are not only flavorful but also tailored to support a diabetic-friendly diet. Packed with wholesome ingredients, these smoothies provide a delightful way to incorporate essential nutrients into your daily routine.

Green Power Smoothie

Ingredients:

- 1 cup kale leaves, stems removed
- 1/2 cup cucumber, peeled and diced
- 1/2 green apple, cored and chopped
- 1/2 cup Greek yogurt (unsweetened)
- 1 tablespoon chia seeds
- 1 cup water or coconut water

Instructions:

1. Combine kale, cucumber, green apple, Greek yogurt, chia seeds, and water in a blender.
2. Blend until smooth and creamy.

3. Pour into a glass and enjoy!

Nutrition Information:

- Calories: 150

- Protein: 8g

- Carbohydrates: 20g

- Fat: 5g

- Fiber: 6g

- Sugar: 10g

- Portion Size: 1 serving

Berry Blast Smoothie

Ingredients:

- 1/2 cup blueberries (fresh or frozen)

- 1/2 cup strawberries, hulled

- 1/2 cup raspberries

- 1/2 banana

- 1/2 cup unsweetened almond milk

- Ice cubes (optional)

Instructions:

1. Combine blueberries, strawberries, raspberries, banana, and almond milk in a blender.
2. Blend until smooth and creamy.
3. Add ice cubes if desired, blend again, and pour into a glass.

Nutrition Information:

- Calories: 120
- Protein: 4g
- Carbohydrates: 25g
- Fat: 2g
- Fiber: 8g
- Sugar: 12g
- Portion Size: 1 serving

Tropical Paradise Smoothie

Ingredients:

- 1/2 cup pineapple chunks
- 1/2 cup mango chunks
- 1/2 banana
- 1/2 cup coconut milk (unsweetened)

- 1 tablespoon flaxseeds

- Ice cubes (optional)

Instructions:

1. Blend pineapple, mango, banana, coconut milk, and flaxseeds until smooth.

2. Add ice cubes if desired and blend again.

3. Pour into a glass and transport yourself to a tropical paradise!

Nutrition Information:

- Calories: 180

- Protein: 5g

- Carbohydrates: 30g

- Fat: 7g

- Fiber: 5g

- Sugar: 15g

- Portion Size: 1 serving

Chocolate Banana Protein Smoothie

Ingredients:

- 1 scoop chocolate protein powder

- 1/2 banana
- 1 tablespoon almond butter
- 1 cup unsweetened almond milk
- 1/2 teaspoon cinnamon
- Ice cubes (optional)

Instructions:

1. Blend chocolate protein powder, banana, almond butter, almond milk, and cinnamon until well combined.
2. Add ice cubes if desired and blend again.
3. Pour into a glass for a satisfying protein boost!

Nutrition Information:

- Calories: 220
- Protein: 20g
- Carbohydrates: 18g
- Fat: 9g
- Fiber: 4g
- Sugar: 6g
- Portion Size: 1 serving

Citrus Sunshine Smoothie

Ingredients:

- 1/2 cup orange segments
- 1/2 cup pineapple chunks
- 1/2 cup Greek yogurt (unsweetened)
- 1 tablespoon honey (optional)
- 1/2 cup water or coconut water
- Ice cubes (optional)

Instructions:

1. Blend orange segments, pineapple, Greek yogurt, honey, and water until smooth.
2. Add ice cubes if desired and blend again.
3. Pour into a glass and bask in the citrusy sunshine flavors!

Nutrition Information:

- Calories: 160
- Protein: 6g
- Carbohydrates: 30g
- Fat: 1g
- Fiber: 4g

- Sugar: 22g

- Portion Size: 1 serving

Kale and Pineapple Smoothie

Ingredients:

- 1 cup kale leaves, stems removed

- 1/2 cup pineapple chunks

- 1/2 banana

- 1/2 cup coconut water

- 1 tablespoon hemp seeds

- Ice cubes (optional)

Instructions:

1. Combine kale, pineapple, banana, coconut water, and hemp seeds in a blender.

2. Blend until smooth and vibrant.

3. Add ice cubes if desired, blend again, and savor the goodness!

Nutrition Information:

- Calories: 140

- Protein: 5g

- Carbohydrates: 25g

- Fat: 4g

- Fiber: 5g

- Sugar: 12g

- Portion Size: 1 serving

Mango Tango Smoothie

Ingredients:

- 1/2 cup mango chunks

- 1/2 cup strawberries, hulled

- 1/2 cup Greek yogurt (unsweetened)

- 1 tablespoon chia seeds

- 1/2 cup water or coconut water

- Ice cubes (optional)

Instructions:

1. Blend mango, strawberries, Greek yogurt, chia seeds, and water until smooth.

2. Incorporate ice cubes if desired and blend again.

3. Pour into a glass and let the mango tango dance on your taste buds!

Nutrition Information:

- Calories: 170

- Protein: 8g

- Carbohydrates: 25g

- Fat: 5g

- Fiber: 7g

- Sugar: 15g

- Portion Size: 1 serving

Peanut Butter and Banana Smoothie

Ingredients:

- 1/2 banana

- 1 tablespoon peanut butter

- 1/2 cup Greek yogurt (unsweetened)

- 1 cup unsweetened almond milk

- 1 tablespoon flaxseeds

- Ice cubes (optional)

Instructions:

1. Blend banana, peanut butter, Greek yogurt, almond milk, and flaxseeds until creamy.

2. Add ice cubes if desired and blend once more.

3. Pour into a glass and relish the classic combo of peanut butter and banana!

Nutrition Information:

- Calories: 220
- Protein: 12g
- Carbohydrates: 20g
- Fat: 10g
- Fiber: 5g
- Sugar: 10g
- Portion Size: 1 serving

Blueberry Almond Butter Smoothie

Ingredients:

- 1/2 cup blueberries (fresh or frozen)
- 1 tablespoon almond butter
- 1/2 cup Greek yogurt (unsweetened)
- 1/2 cup almond milk
- 1 tablespoon chia seeds
- Ice cubes (optional)

Instructions:

1. Blend blueberries, almond butter, Greek yogurt, almond milk, and chia seeds until smooth.
2. If desired, add ice cubes and blend again.
3. Pour into a glass and enjoy the delightful blend of blueberries and almond butter!

Nutrition Information:

- Calories: 180
- Protein: 8g
- Carbohydrates: 22g
- Fat: 8g
- Fiber: 6g
- Sugar: 14g
- Portion Size: 1 serving

Spinach and Apple Smoothie

Ingredients:

- 1 cup spinach leaves
- 1/2 green apple, cored and chopped
- 1/2 banana
- 1/2 cup Greek yogurt (unsweetened)

- 1/2 cup water or coconut water
- Ice cubes (optional)

Instructions:

1. Blend spinach, green apple, banana, Greek yogurt, and water until smooth.
2. Include ice cubes if desired, blend again, and relish the vibrant green goodness.
3. Pour into a glass and enjoy this nutrient-packed smoothie!

Nutrition Information:

- Calories: 130
- Protein: 6g
- Carbohydrates: 25g
- Fat: 2g
- Fiber: 5g
- Sugar: 15g
- Portion Size: 1 serving

Chia Seed and Strawberry Smoothie

Ingredients:

- 1/2 cup strawberries, hulled
- 1/2 banana
- 1 tablespoon chia seeds
- 1/2 cup Greek yogurt (unsweetened)
- 1/2 cup almond milk
- Ice cubes (optional)

Instructions:

1. Blend strawberries, banana, chia seeds, Greek yogurt, and almond milk until smooth.
2. Add ice cubes if desired, blend again, and indulge in this chia-packed delight.
3. Pour into a glass and relish the combination of strawberries and chia seeds!

Nutrition Information:

- Calories: 150
- Protein: 7g
- Carbohydrates: 20g
- Fat: 6g

- Fiber: 8g
- Sugar: 12g
- Portion Size: 1 serving

Coffee and Oat Smoothie

Ingredients:

- 1/2 cup brewed coffee, cooled
- 1/4 cup rolled oats
- 1/2 banana
- 1/2 cup Greek yogurt (unsweetened)
- 1/2 cup almond milk
- Ice cubes (optional)

Instructions:

1. Blend brewed coffee, rolled oats, banana, Greek yogurt, and almond milk until well combined.
2. If desired, add ice cubes and blend again for a refreshing kick.
3. Pour into a glass and savor the unique blend of coffee and oats!

Nutrition Information:

- Calories: 160
- Protein: 7g
- Carbohydrates: 25g
- Fat: 5g
- Fiber: 5g
- Sugar: 8g
- Portion Size: 1 serving

Peachy Keen Protein Smoothie

Ingredients:

- 1/2 cup peaches, sliced
- 1 scoop vanilla protein powder
- 1/2 cup Greek yogurt (unsweetened)
- 1/2 cup almond milk
- 1 tablespoon flaxseeds
- Ice cubes (optional)

Instructions:

1. Blend peaches, vanilla protein powder, Greek yogurt, almond milk, and flaxseeds until smooth.

2. Include ice cubes if desired, blend again, and revel in the peachy protein goodness.

3. Pour into a glass and enjoy this protein-packed peach delight!

Nutrition Information:

- Calories: 200
- Protein: 20g
- Carbohydrates: 18g
- Fat: 7g
- Fiber: 4g
- Sugar: 12g
- Portion Size: 1 serving

Avocado Spinach Smoothie

Ingredients:

- 1/2 avocado, peeled and pitted
- 1 cup spinach leaves
- 1/2 banana
- 1/2 cup coconut water
- 1 tablespoon hemp seeds
- Ice cubes (optional)

Instructions:

1. Blend avocado, spinach, banana, coconut water, and hemp seeds until creamy.

2. If desired, add ice cubes and blend again for a refreshing touch.

3. Pour into a glass and savor the creamy blend of avocado and spinach!

Nutrition Information:

- Calories: 180
- Protein: 8g
- Carbohydrates: 22g
- Fat: 9g
- Fiber: 6g
- Sugar: 10g
- Portion Size: 1 serving

Mixed Berry Coconut Water Smoothie

Ingredients:

- 1/2 cup mixed berries (strawberries, blueberries, raspberries)
- 1/2 cup coconut water
- 1/2 banana
- 1/2 cup Greek yogurt (unsweetened)
- 1 tablespoon chia seeds
- Ice cubes (optional)

Instructions:

1. Blend mixed berries, coconut water, banana, Greek yogurt, and chia seeds until smooth.
2. Add ice cubes if desired, blend again, and delight in the refreshing mixed berry goodness.
3. Pour into a glass and enjoy this antioxidant-rich smoothie!

Nutrition Information:

- Calories: 140
- Protein: 7g

- Carbohydrates: 25g
- Fat: 4g
- Fiber: 8g
- Sugar: 15g
- Portion Size: 1 serving

CONCLUSION

In concluding the "Easy Diabetic Cookbook for Beginners," we hope this culinary guide serves as more than just a compilation of recipes; rather, a tool to empower your journey towards a healthier, tastier lifestyle despite diabetes. By embracing the carefully curated meal plans and diverse recipes, you embark on a flavorful adventure that not only caters to your dietary needs but also celebrates the joy of eating.

This cookbook is not just about restrictions; it's a celebration of culinary creativity within the boundaries of a diabetic-friendly diet. The 30-day meal plan sets the stage for a systematic and sustainable approach to managing your nutrition, providing a roadmap to balanced, delicious meals throughout the month.

The breakfast, lunch, and dinner recipes encompass a wide array of flavors, textures, and nutritional benefits. From the hearty Nutty Oatmeal Delight to the refreshing Grilled Chicken Salad with Lemon Vinaigrette, each dish is crafted with both taste and health in mind. The snacks, desserts, and smoothies offer delightful treats without compromising on nutritional value, proving that indulgence can indeed be guilt-free.

Remember, this cookbook is not just about what you can't eat; it's about discovering the abundance of delicious options that are readily available. Embrace the journey of trying new ingredients, experimenting with flavors, and finding joy in the kitchen. Through mindful choices and the culinary exploration offered in these pages, you are not just managing diabetes; you are thriving with it.

As you navigate the chapters and savor the recipes, we hope this cookbook becomes a trusted companion on your path to wellness. May it inspire creativity in your kitchen, foster a love for wholesome ingredients, and, most importantly, remind you that eating well with diabetes is not a compromise but a delicious adventure. Here's to health, happiness, and the joy of nourishing your body with every delectable bite. Cheers to your vibrant and flavorful diabetic journey!